Publisher Inform

Before reading the book, please read the disclaimer.

For permissions, inquiries, or other correspondence:
drmedhealth.com@gmail.com

For more information, please visit.

www.DrMedHealth.com

Disclaimer

The content of this book is a work of fiction. Names, characters, places, medical scenarios, and incidents are either the product of the author's imagination or are used fictitiously. Any resemblance to actual persons, living or dead, real-life medical events, organizations, or institutions is purely coincidental.

The medical procedures, treatments, and conditions described are for narrative purposes only and should not be interpreted as professional advice. Readers are advised not to use the medical information presented in this book as a substitute for consulting healthcare professionals or seeking proper medical care.

Neither the author, Dr. Nilesh Panchal, nor the publisher, **DrMedHealth**, assumes any responsibility for actions taken based on the information contained within these novels. Any opinions expressed in the book are solely those of the author and do not represent the views of any affiliated institutions or organizations.

What is Meningitis, and What Are Its Main Types?

Meningitis is a medical condition that strikes fear into the hearts of many because of its potential severity and life-altering consequences. At its core, meningitis is the inflammation of the meninges—the protective membranes that envelop the brain and spinal cord. These membranes, along with the cerebrospinal fluid (CSF) they contain, act as a cushion to shield the central nervous system from trauma and infection. When the meninges become inflamed, the repercussions can range from mild discomfort to severe neurological damage, and in some cases, death.

Understanding Meningitis

The term "meningitis" derives from the Greek word *meninx*, meaning membrane, and the suffix *-itis*, which signifies inflammation. While the condition may be caused by various factors, it is most commonly the result of an infection. The infection triggers an immune response, leading to inflammation that can cause increased pressure in the brain, disruption of normal neurological function, and other systemic effects. Meningitis is a global health concern, impacting people of all ages, although certain populations, such as infants, the elderly, and immunocompromised individuals, are particularly vulnerable.

The disease's progression can be swift, making early recognition and treatment critical. The hallmark symptoms include a sudden onset of fever, severe headache, neck stiffness, nausea, vomiting, sensitivity to light (photophobia), and confusion. In infants, the presentation may include irritability, poor feeding, a bulging soft spot on the head (fontanel), and an abnormal cry. Recognizing these signs promptly can make the difference between a full recovery and devastating complications.

The Different Types of Meningitis

Meningitis is not a one-size-fits-all condition; it has various forms, each with distinct causes, symptoms, and treatment approaches. Broadly, meningitis can be classified into infectious and non-infectious categories. The infectious forms are further divided into bacterial, viral, fungal, and parasitic meningitis, while non-infectious meningitis arises from causes such as autoimmune diseases, cancer, or certain medications.

1. Bacterial Meningitis

Bacterial meningitis is the most severe and potentially life-threatening form of meningitis. It occurs when bacteria invade the bloodstream and cross the blood-brain barrier, infecting the meninges. The infection can progress rapidly, often within hours, necessitating immediate medical attention.

Common Causes

Several bacterial species are responsible for meningitis, with the most common being:

- **Streptococcus pneumoniae (pneumococcal meningitis):** This is the leading cause of bacterial meningitis in adults and children. It is often associated with infections like pneumonia, sinusitis, or ear infections.
- **Neisseria meningitidis (meningococcal meningitis):** Known for causing outbreaks, this type is highly contagious and can spread through respiratory droplets. It often affects adolescents and young adults.
- **Haemophilus influenzae type b (Hib):** Once a leading cause of meningitis in children, the Hib vaccine has significantly reduced its prevalence.
- **Listeria monocytogenes:** This bacterium can cause meningitis in newborns, pregnant women, and individuals with weakened immune systems. It is often linked to contaminated food.
- **Escherichia coli and Group B Streptococcus:** Common causes of meningitis in newborns, typically acquired during childbirth.

Symptoms and Complications

Bacterial meningitis symptoms typically include high fever, severe headache, and neck stiffness. As

6

the infection progresses, it may lead to seizures, hearing loss, or cognitive deficits. In severe cases, it can result in septic shock, coma, or death.

Treatment

Bacterial meningitis requires urgent treatment with intravenous antibiotics and, in some cases, corticosteroids to reduce inflammation. Supportive care, such as fluid management and monitoring for complications, is also essential.

2. Viral Meningitis

Viral meningitis, also known as aseptic meningitis, is the most common form of the disease. Although it is typically less severe than bacterial meningitis, it can still cause significant discomfort and health challenges.

Common Causes

Viral meningitis is caused by a range of viruses, including:

- **Enteroviruses:** These viruses account for most cases, particularly in late summer and early fall.
- **Herpes simplex virus (HSV):** Both HSV-1 (commonly associated with cold sores) and HSV-2 (linked to genital herpes) can cause meningitis.

- **Varicella-zoster virus (VZV):** This virus, responsible for chickenpox and shingles, can lead to meningitis.
- **HIV:** In some cases, the early stages of HIV infection can present as viral meningitis.
- **Arboviruses:** Transmitted by mosquitoes or ticks, these viruses include West Nile virus and St. Louis encephalitis virus.

Symptoms and Complications

Symptoms of viral meningitis are similar to bacterial meningitis but are usually milder. Fever, headache, and neck stiffness are common, though seizures and neurological complications are rare.

Treatment

Most cases of viral meningitis resolve on their own within 7–10 days, requiring only supportive care such as rest, hydration, and pain management. Antiviral medications may be prescribed for meningitis caused by herpes viruses.

3. Fungal Meningitis

Fungal meningitis is a rare but serious form of the disease. It occurs when fungal spores enter the bloodstream and spread to the meninges. This type of meningitis is most common in individuals with weakened immune systems, such as those with HIV/AIDS or undergoing chemotherapy.

Common Causes

- **Cryptococcus:** This fungus is a leading cause of fungal meningitis, particularly in people with HIV/AIDS.
- **Candida:** Commonly known for causing yeast infections, Candida can also lead to meningitis in hospitalized patients.
- **Histoplasma and Blastomyces:** These fungi are found in soil and bird droppings and can cause meningitis in endemic regions.

Symptoms and Complications

Fungal meningitis symptoms develop gradually, often over weeks, and include headache, fever, nausea, and altered mental status. Without treatment, it can lead to severe neurological damage.

Treatment

Treatment involves prolonged courses of antifungal medications, such as amphotericin B and fluconazole. Early diagnosis and treatment are critical for improving outcomes.

4. Parasitic Meningitis

Parasitic meningitis is an uncommon form of the disease, typically caused by parasites found in contaminated water or food. One of the most notorious parasites is *Naegleria fowleri*, also known as the "brain-eating amoeba," which causes primary amebic meningoencephalitis (PAM), a rare but almost universally fatal condition.

Common Causes

- **Naegleria fowleri:** Found in warm freshwater, this parasite can infect individuals swimming in contaminated water.
- **Angiostrongylus cantonensis (rat lungworm):** This parasite is found in certain parts of Asia and the Pacific and is transmitted through contaminated food.
- **Toxoplasma gondii:** Typically associated with cats and contaminated meat, this parasite can occasionally cause meningitis in immunocompromised individuals.

Symptoms and Complications

Parasitic meningitis often presents with a rapid onset of severe headache, fever, vomiting, and neurological symptoms. Prognosis varies depending on the specific parasite involved.

Treatment

Treatment depends on the specific parasite and may include antiparasitic medications, supportive care, and in some cases, experimental therapies.

5. Non-Infectious Meningitis

Non-infectious meningitis is caused by factors other than infections, such as autoimmune disorders, cancer, medications, or trauma. While it does not involve infectious pathogens, it can still cause significant health issues.

Common Causes

- **Autoimmune diseases:** Conditions like lupus or sarcoidosis can trigger inflammation of the meninges.
- **Cancer:** Metastatic cancer cells can invade the meninges, leading to a condition known as carcinomatous meningitis.
- **Medications:** Certain drugs, such as nonsteroidal anti-inflammatory drugs (NSAIDs) or intravenous immunoglobulin (IVIG), have been associated with meningitis.
- **Trauma:** Head injuries or neurosurgical procedures can result in meningitis.

Symptoms and Complications

Symptoms mimic those of infectious meningitis and include headache, fever, and neck stiffness. Complications depend on the underlying cause and severity of the inflammation.

Treatment

Treatment focuses on addressing the underlying cause, such as immunosuppressive therapy for autoimmune diseases or discontinuing the offending medication.

Meningitis is a complex and multifaceted disease with diverse causes and manifestations. Understanding its types and their distinguishing features is the first step toward effective prevention, diagnosis, and treatment. The subsequent chapters of this book will delve deeper into these aspects, equipping readers with the knowledge needed to recognize, manage, and prevent this serious condition.

What Are the Common Causes of Meningitis, and How Is It Transmitted?

Meningitis, a potentially life-threatening condition, arises when the protective membranes surrounding the brain and spinal cord—the meninges—become inflamed. Understanding the causes and modes of transmission of meningitis is crucial to preventing its spread and managing its impact on individuals and communities. This chapter delves into the wide array of pathogens responsible for meningitis and the mechanisms through which they infiltrate the human body, offering a comprehensive view of this complex disease.

Understanding the Causes of Meningitis

The causes of meningitis are diverse and multifaceted, but they share a common thread: an invasion of the meninges by infectious agents or, in some cases, non-infectious triggers. The most frequent culprits include bacteria, viruses, fungi, and parasites. Each of these agents has unique characteristics, behaviors, and pathways of infection. Additionally, meningitis can occasionally result from non-infectious factors such as autoimmune diseases, cancer, or medications.

Bacterial Causes of Meningitis

Bacterial meningitis is one of the most severe forms of the disease, characterized by rapid onset and the potential for significant complications, including neurological damage and death. Several bacteria are known to cause meningitis, each with distinct epidemiology and transmission pathways.

1. Neisseria meningitidis (Meningococcus)

One of the most common causes of bacterial meningitis, *Neisseria meningitidis*, is a gram-negative bacterium that exists in multiple serogroups (A, B, C, W, X, and Y). Meningococcal meningitis often strikes in outbreaks, particularly in crowded settings such as college dormitories, military barracks, and refugee camps.

- **Transmission:** *N. meningitidis* spreads through respiratory droplets, making close contact with an infected person or carrier a significant risk factor. Activities such as coughing, sneezing, kissing, or sharing utensils facilitate its transmission.
- **Pathogenesis:** Once inside the body, the bacteria can colonize the nasopharynx. In some individuals, it invades the bloodstream and crosses the blood-brain barrier, leading to meningitis.

2. Streptococcus pneumoniae (Pneumococcus)

Streptococcus pneumoniae is another leading cause of bacterial meningitis, particularly in infants, young children, and the elderly. This gram-positive bacterium is also associated with other infections such as pneumonia, sinusitis, and otitis media.

- **Transmission:** Pneumococcal meningitis is typically acquired through respiratory droplets. The bacteria can exist harmlessly in the nasopharynx of healthy carriers but may become invasive under certain conditions, such as a weakened immune system.
- **Pathogenesis:** Following entry into the bloodstream, *S. pneumoniae* can penetrate the meninges, causing intense inflammation.

3. Haemophilus influenzae (Hib)

Before the advent of the Hib vaccine, *Haemophilus influenzae* type b was a common cause of bacterial meningitis in children. While cases have declined significantly in vaccinated populations, it remains a concern in areas with low vaccine coverage.

- **Transmission:** Like other respiratory pathogens, Hib spreads through respiratory droplets or direct contact with secretions from an infected individual.

- **Pathogenesis:** Hib can cause upper respiratory tract infections, which may progress to invasive diseases like meningitis in susceptible individuals.

4. Listeria monocytogenes

This bacterium is an uncommon cause of meningitis, primarily affecting newborns, pregnant women, older adults, and immunocompromised individuals. It is often associated with contaminated food.

- **Transmission:** *Listeria monocytogenes* is transmitted through the consumption of contaminated food products, such as unpasteurized dairy, deli meats, and raw vegetables.
- **Pathogenesis:** After entering the gastrointestinal tract, the bacterium can invade the bloodstream and cross the blood-brain barrier, causing meningitis.

5. Group B Streptococcus (GBS) and Escherichia coli

These bacteria are leading causes of meningitis in newborns, often transmitted during childbirth.

- **Transmission:** Neonates acquire GBS or *E. coli* during delivery from an infected mother's birth canal or through hospital environments.
- **Pathogenesis:** Both bacteria can rapidly spread through the bloodstream to the

central nervous system, causing severe inflammation.

Viral Causes of Meningitis

Viral meningitis, also known as aseptic meningitis, is the most common form of the disease. While generally less severe than bacterial meningitis, it can still cause significant discomfort and prolonged recovery in some individuals. Many different viruses are implicated in its development.

1. Enteroviruses

Enteroviruses, such as Coxsackievirus and Echovirus, are responsible for most cases of viral meningitis. They are particularly active in late summer and early fall.

- **Transmission:** These viruses are transmitted through the fecal-oral route, contaminated water, or respiratory droplets.
- **Pathogenesis:** After entering the body, enteroviruses replicate in the gastrointestinal tract and can spread to the central nervous system via the bloodstream.

2. Herpes Simplex Virus (HSV)

Both HSV-1 (commonly causing cold sores) and HSV-2 (linked to genital herpes) can cause viral meningitis. HSV meningitis may recur in some individuals.

- **Transmission:** HSV is transmitted through direct contact with infected bodily fluids or lesions.
- **Pathogenesis:** The virus can remain dormant in the nervous system and reactivate, occasionally affecting the meninges.

3. Varicella-Zoster Virus (VZV)

This virus, known for causing chickenpox and shingles, can also lead to meningitis.

- **Transmission:** VZV spreads through respiratory droplets or direct contact with the fluid from chickenpox or shingles blisters.
- **Pathogenesis:** Following initial infection, the virus can reactivate from the dorsal root ganglia and affect the meninges.

4. Other Viruses

Other viruses, such as HIV, mumps virus, and arboviruses like West Nile virus, can also cause meningitis. Arboviruses are transmitted through vectors like mosquitoes or ticks.

Fungal Causes of Meningitis

Fungal meningitis is rare and generally affects individuals with compromised immune systems, such as those with HIV/AIDS, cancer, or organ transplants. It is often chronic and requires long-term treatment.

1. Cryptococcus

Cryptococcal meningitis, caused by *Cryptococcus neoformans* or *Cryptococcus gattii*, is one of the most common forms of fungal meningitis.

- **Transmission:** Fungal spores are inhaled from the environment, typically from soil or bird droppings.
- **Pathogenesis:** The fungus spreads from the lungs to the bloodstream and crosses the blood-brain barrier, leading to meningitis.

2. Candida

While typically associated with bloodstream infections, *Candida* species can occasionally cause meningitis, particularly in hospitalized patients.

3. Endemic Fungi

Fungi like *Histoplasma capsulatum* and *Coccidioides* can cause meningitis in individuals living in endemic regions.

Parasitic Causes of Meningitis

Parasitic meningitis is rare but can be devastating. It includes conditions such as primary amebic meningoencephalitis (PAM) caused by *Naegleria fowleri*.

- **Transmission:** Parasites are often transmitted through contaminated water or food. *Naegleria fowleri* infects individuals swimming in warm, untreated freshwater.
- **Pathogenesis:** Once in the nasal passages, the parasite migrates to the brain, causing rapid and fatal inflammation.

Non-Infectious Causes of Meningitis

Non-infectious meningitis results from non-pathogenic triggers such as autoimmune diseases, cancer, medications, or trauma. Though less common, it presents with symptoms similar to infectious meningitis.

- **Examples of Causes:**
  - Autoimmune diseases like lupus
  - Cancer spreading to the meninges (carcinomatous meningitis)
  - Medications causing drug-induced meningitis

How Meningitis Is Transmitted

The transmission of meningitis depends on the causative agent. Most forms of meningitis involve person-to-person spread or exposure to environmental sources.

1. Respiratory Droplets

Bacterial and viral meningitis caused by pathogens like *Neisseria meningitidis*, *Streptococcus pneumoniae*, and enteroviruses often spread through respiratory droplets. Coughing, sneezing, or close contact facilitates this transmission.

2. Fecal-Oral Route

Enteroviruses and some parasitic causes of meningitis spread through the ingestion of contaminated water or food.

3. Bloodborne Transmission

Pathogens like *Listeria monocytogenes* and HIV can enter the bloodstream and subsequently invade the central nervous system.

4. Direct Contact

Close contact with infected bodily fluids, such as saliva, nasal secretions, or blister fluid, is another mode of transmission for pathogens like HSV and VZV.

5. Vector-Borne

Arboviruses are transmitted through insect vectors like mosquitoes or ticks.

6. Environmental Exposure

Fungi and parasites are typically acquired from environmental sources, such as contaminated soil, bird droppings, or warm freshwater bodies.

Preventing Transmission

Understanding the modes of transmission is crucial for preventing meningitis. Vaccination, proper hygiene practices, safe food handling, and public health measures during outbreaks are vital tools in reducing the incidence of this disease.

The causes and transmission pathways of meningitis are as varied as the disease itself. By identifying the responsible pathogens and their routes of spread, we can better combat this complex condition through targeted prevention and treatment strategies. In the following chapters, we will explore how to recognize the signs and symptoms of meningitis and the diagnostic tools used to confirm its presence.

What Are the Key Signs and Symptoms of Meningitis in Children, Adults, and the Elderly?

Meningitis, an inflammation of the protective membranes surrounding the brain and spinal cord, presents a wide range of symptoms. These symptoms vary significantly based on the age of the patient, the causative agent, and the severity of the infection. Early recognition of these signs is critical, as meningitis can progress rapidly and lead to severe complications or death without prompt medical intervention. This chapter explores the key signs and symptoms of meningitis across different age groups—children, adults, and the elderly—highlighting the unique ways it manifests in each population.

Understanding Meningitis Symptoms

Meningitis symptoms arise due to the inflammation of the meninges and the immune response to the invading pathogen. This inflammation can increase intracranial pressure, impair neurological function, and cause systemic illness. While some symptoms, such as fever, headache, and neck stiffness, are considered classic indicators of meningitis, others can be subtler and harder to detect, especially in vulnerable populations like infants and the elderly.

The hallmark symptoms of meningitis include:

- **Fever:** A sudden, high-grade fever is often the first sign of an infection.
- **Severe headache:** This headache is persistent and unrelieved by over-the-counter medications.
- **Neck stiffness:** A reduced ability to move the neck, especially difficulty bending it forward, is a key diagnostic sign.
- **Nausea and vomiting:** These symptoms are common due to increased intracranial pressure.
- **Photophobia:** Sensitivity to light, which exacerbates discomfort and headache.
- **Confusion or altered mental status:** Difficulty concentrating, confusion, or outright unresponsiveness can occur as the brain becomes inflamed.
- **Seizures:** In severe cases, meningitis can trigger seizures due to irritation of the brain tissue.
- **Skin rash:** In certain types, particularly meningococcal meningitis, a distinctive purplish rash may appear.

These symptoms are not universal, and their presentation can vary based on age and individual health conditions.

Symptoms in Children and Infants

Children, especially infants, are at a higher risk of meningitis due to their immature immune systems. However, the symptoms in this age group can be vague and difficult to recognize, making diagnosis particularly challenging.

1. Symptoms in Infants (0–12 months)

In infants, meningitis may present with non-specific symptoms that mimic common illnesses. This can lead to delays in seeking medical attention. Key symptoms include:

- **Fever or hypothermia:** While fever is a common sign, some infants may exhibit a drop in body temperature (hypothermia).
- **Irritability or inconsolable crying:** Persistent crying that worsens when the baby is held is a red flag.
- **Poor feeding:** Infants with meningitis may refuse to feed or have difficulty breastfeeding.
- **Lethargy or difficulty waking:** A lack of energy or excessive sleepiness is a concerning symptom.
- **Bulging fontanel:** The soft spot on an infant's head may appear swollen due to increased intracranial pressure.

- **Stiff body or floppy limbs:** Some infants may have rigid muscles, while others may appear weak and floppy.
- **Abnormal movements:** Seizures or jerky movements can occur in severe cases.

2. Symptoms in Young Children (1–5 years)

Young children may be better able to express discomfort, but their symptoms can still overlap with those of other illnesses:

- **Fever and headache:** These are common but can be attributed to other childhood infections.
- **Neck pain or stiffness:** A reluctance to move the neck is more noticeable in older children.
- **Nausea and vomiting:** These are common and may be mistaken for a gastrointestinal illness.
- **Aversion to bright light:** Photophobia can be expressed as discomfort in well-lit environments.
- **Behavioral changes:** Irritability, confusion, or disinterest in usual activities may indicate neurological involvement.
- **Rashes:** A purplish or blotchy rash should immediately raise suspicion of meningococcal meningitis.

Symptoms in Adults

In adults, the symptoms of meningitis are typically more recognizable and align closely with the classic triad of fever, headache, and neck stiffness. However, the severity and progression can vary based on the individual's overall health and the type of meningitis.

1. Classic Symptoms

- **Fever:** A high-grade fever that develops rapidly is common.
- **Severe headache:** The headache is often described as the worst the person has ever experienced.
- **Neck stiffness:** Difficulty or pain in bending the neck forward is a critical diagnostic clue.
- **Nausea and vomiting:** These symptoms often accompany the headache.
- **Photophobia:** Adults may complain of sensitivity to light, which worsens their headache.

2. Neurological Symptoms

As the disease progresses, adults may exhibit neurological symptoms, including:

- **Confusion or altered mental status:** Trouble concentrating, memory loss, or unresponsiveness may occur.

- **Seizures:** These can result from irritation of the brain tissue or increased intracranial pressure.
- **Sleepiness or difficulty waking:** Drowsiness or a tendency to fall asleep easily is a warning sign of severe meningitis.
- **Coma:** In advanced cases, meningitis can lead to a coma.

3. Additional Signs

- **Skin rash:** Meningococcal meningitis can cause a petechial or purpuric rash that does not fade when pressed.
- **Cold extremities or rapid breathing:** These may indicate septicemia associated with meningitis.

Symptoms in the Elderly

Meningitis in the elderly often presents atypically, making diagnosis particularly challenging. The immune response in older adults may be blunted, leading to subtle or non-classic symptoms.

1. Atypical Presentation

- **Low-grade fever or absence of fever:** Unlike younger populations, the elderly may not develop a high fever.

- **Lethargy or altered mental status:**
  Confusion, disorientation, or a sudden
  decline in cognitive function may be the
  only noticeable symptoms.
- **Headache and neck stiffness:** These
  symptoms may be milder or absent in older
  adults.
- **Falls or unsteadiness:** Difficulty walking or
  frequent falls may be an early sign of
  neurological involvement.

2. Severe Symptoms

- **Seizures:** Though less common, seizures
  can occur in severe cases.
- **Coma:** In advanced meningitis, elderly
  patients are at higher risk of slipping into a
  coma due to delayed recognition and
  treatment.

Symptom Differences by Causative Agent

The causative agent of meningitis can influence the
symptom profile:

1. Bacterial Meningitis

- Symptoms tend to develop rapidly, often
  within hours to days.
- Severe headache, fever, and neck stiffness
  are hallmark symptoms.

- Neurological symptoms such as seizures and confusion are common.
- Meningococcal meningitis may present with a purplish rash.

2. Viral Meningitis

- Symptoms are generally milder and may include fever, headache, and photophobia.
- Neurological complications are rare.
- Most cases resolve without specific treatment.

3. Fungal Meningitis

- Symptoms develop gradually over weeks and may mimic chronic illnesses.
- Headache, fever, and lethargy are common.
- Neurological symptoms may appear in advanced stages.

4. Parasitic Meningitis

- Symptoms depend on the specific parasite but often include rapid onset of fever, headache, and neurological decline.
- Primary amebic meningoencephalitis caused by *Naegleria fowleri* is characterized by rapid progression and high fatality rates.

5. Non-Infectious Meningitis

- Symptoms vary based on the underlying cause (e.g., autoimmune disease or cancer).
- Fever and headache are common but may be less pronounced.

Complications of Delayed Recognition

Delays in recognizing and treating meningitis can lead to severe complications, including:

- **Hearing loss:** Damage to the auditory nerves is a common long-term effect.
- **Seizures:** Persistent seizures may develop as a result of brain damage.
- **Cognitive deficits:** Memory loss, difficulty concentrating, and other neurological issues can persist.
- **Hydrocephalus:** Accumulation of cerebrospinal fluid can lead to increased intracranial pressure.
- **Death:** Without timely treatment, bacterial meningitis, in particular, has a high mortality rate.

The signs and symptoms of meningitis vary widely based on age, health status, and the underlying cause. While classic symptoms like fever, headache, and neck stiffness are common, recognizing the subtler signs in infants, the elderly, and immunocompromised individuals is critical. Understanding these variations can lead to earlier diagnosis, prompt treatment, and better outcomes. In the next chapter, we will explore the diagnostic tools and techniques used to confirm meningitis, providing insight into the essential steps that follow symptom recognition.

What Are the Potential Complications of Untreated Meningitis?

Meningitis is a medical emergency that demands immediate attention. When left untreated, it can lead to devastating complications, some of which are irreversible. The condition affects the brain and spinal cord—two of the most critical components of the central nervous system (CNS)—and its complications can disrupt the body's normal functioning in both the short and long term. Understanding these complications is vital for appreciating the seriousness of meningitis and the necessity of early diagnosis and treatment.

This chapter explores the various short-term and long-term effects of untreated meningitis, ranging from brain damage and hearing loss to life-threatening conditions like hydrocephalus, seizures, and death. These outcomes not only impact the patient but also have a profound effect on families, caregivers, and society.

The Mechanisms of Meningitis-Related Complications

The complications of meningitis are largely the result of the inflammation it causes in the meninges and surrounding tissues. When the body's immune system responds to an infection, it triggers an inflammatory process aimed at eradicating the pathogen. However, in the confined space of the cranial cavity, this inflammation can cause increased intracranial pressure, tissue damage, and disruption of normal blood flow to the brain. These effects, combined with the direct damage caused by the invading pathogens, lead to the complications described below.

Short-Term Complications

Short-term complications of meningitis typically emerge during the acute phase of the illness. These complications can rapidly worsen and may require immediate medical intervention.

1. Increased Intracranial Pressure

One of the most immediate dangers of meningitis is increased intracranial pressure (ICP). The inflammation of the meninges leads to swelling, which compresses the brain tissue within the skull.

- **Symptoms:** Severe headache, nausea, vomiting, and altered mental status are common symptoms of increased ICP. In infants, a bulging fontanel (soft spot) may be observed.

- **Consequences:** If left unaddressed, elevated ICP can lead to herniation, where brain tissue is forced downward into the spinal canal, causing coma or death.

2. Seizures

Seizures are a frequent complication of untreated meningitis, especially bacterial meningitis. The irritation and inflammation of the brain tissue trigger abnormal electrical activity.

- **Acute Seizures:** These may occur in the early stages of meningitis and are often generalized, affecting the entire body.
- **Status Epilepticus:** A prolonged seizure lasting more than five minutes or multiple seizures without recovery in between can occur and is a medical emergency.
- **Long-Term Risk:** Some patients develop epilepsy as a result of the brain damage caused by prolonged seizures during meningitis.

3. Septicemia (Blood Poisoning)

In some cases, the bacteria responsible for meningitis can enter the bloodstream, causing septicemia. This condition is particularly associated with meningococcal meningitis.

- **Symptoms:** Rapid heart rate, low blood pressure, cold extremities, and a distinctive purpuric rash (dark purple spots) that does not fade under pressure.

- **Consequences:** Septicemia can progress to septic shock, a life-threatening condition characterized by multi-organ failure.

4. Acute Neurological Deficits

During the acute phase, patients may experience neurological deficits such as confusion, drowsiness, or difficulty speaking or moving. These symptoms often result from increased ICP or localized damage caused by the infection.

Long-Term Complications

For patients who survive the acute phase of meningitis, long-term complications can persist, sometimes for life. These complications often result from permanent damage to the brain, spinal cord, or sensory organs.

1. Brain Damage

Brain damage is one of the most severe and life-altering complications of meningitis. It occurs due to the combined effects of inflammation, increased ICP, and reduced blood flow to brain tissues.

- **Cognitive Impairment:** Survivors may experience memory loss, difficulty concentrating, or reduced problem-solving abilities.

- **Behavioral Changes:** Personality changes, emotional instability, and increased irritability are common in individuals with brain damage.
- **Motor Impairments:** Damage to specific brain regions can lead to weakness, paralysis, or coordination issues.

2. Hearing Loss

Hearing loss is a well-documented complication of meningitis, particularly bacterial meningitis. The infection and inflammation can damage the cochlea, auditory nerve, or other structures in the inner ear.

- **Severity:** Hearing loss can range from mild to profound and may affect one or both ears.
- **Impact on Children:** Hearing loss in children can delay language development and affect educational outcomes.
- **Management:** In some cases, cochlear implants or hearing aids can restore partial hearing.

3. Vision Problems

The inflammation associated with meningitis can also affect the eyes and optic nerves, leading to vision problems.

- **Blurred Vision:** Swelling of the optic nerve (papilledema) can cause blurred or double vision.
- **Blindness:** Severe cases may result in partial or complete loss of vision.

4. Hydrocephalus

Hydrocephalus, or the accumulation of cerebrospinal fluid (CSF) in the brain, is a potential complication of meningitis. This occurs when the normal flow of CSF is obstructed by scarring or inflammation.

- **Symptoms:** Headache, nausea, difficulty walking, and in severe cases, coma.
- **Treatment:** A shunt may be surgically inserted to drain excess fluid and relieve pressure.

5. Developmental Delays in Children

Children who survive meningitis may experience developmental delays due to the effects of brain damage.

- **Learning Disabilities:** Difficulty with reading, writing, or mathematics may emerge in school-aged children.
- **Motor Delays:** Some children may struggle with gross and fine motor skills.

- **Social and Emotional Challenges:**
  Behavioral issues and difficulties in social
  interaction can also arise.

6. Chronic Headaches

Survivors of meningitis often report persistent
headaches, which may be caused by residual
inflammation, scarring, or increased sensitivity to
pain.

- **Management:** Medications, physical
  therapy, and lifestyle changes may help
  manage chronic headaches.

7. Psychological and Emotional Effects

The experience of severe illness and its aftermath
can take a toll on a survivor's mental health.

- **Anxiety and Depression:** Many patients
  struggle with anxiety, depression, or post-
  traumatic stress disorder (PTSD) after
  recovery.
- **Impact on Caregivers:** Family members
  and caregivers may also experience
  emotional distress, particularly if the patient
  has severe disabilities.

Fatal Outcomes

For many patients, the complications of untreated meningitis can be fatal. The mortality rate varies depending on the type of meningitis and the availability of timely treatment.

1. Death Due to Bacterial Meningitis

Bacterial meningitis has the highest mortality rate among the types of meningitis, with some studies reporting rates as high as 20–30% in untreated cases.

- **Causes of Death:** Septic shock, brain herniation, or multi-organ failure are common causes of death.

2. Death in Viral Meningitis

While viral meningitis is generally less severe, certain forms—such as those caused by herpes simplex virus or arboviruses—can be life-threatening if not treated promptly.

The Broader Impact of Meningitis Complications

The complications of meningitis extend beyond the individual, affecting families, healthcare systems, and society as a whole.

1. Economic Burden

The costs associated with prolonged hospital stays, rehabilitation, and lifelong care can be substantial.

- **For Families:** Many families face financial hardship due to medical expenses and lost income.
- **For Healthcare Systems:** Meningitis outbreaks place a significant strain on healthcare resources.

2. Social and Educational Impact

Survivors, particularly children, may require special education services or accommodations in school. This can impact their ability to achieve their full potential.

3. Psychological Toll

The emotional and psychological impact on survivors and their families is often profound, requiring ongoing support and counseling.

Prevention and Early Treatment: The Key to Avoiding Complications

The devastating complications of meningitis highlight the importance of prevention and early intervention. Vaccination remains the most effective tool in reducing the incidence of bacterial meningitis caused by *Haemophilus influenzae* type b (Hib), *Neisseria meningitidis*, and *Streptococcus pneumoniae*. Public health measures, including education about hygiene and prompt medical care for infections, also play a critical role.

Meningitis is a formidable disease with potentially life-altering complications. From brain damage and sensory impairments to the ultimate loss of life, the consequences of untreated meningitis underscore the need for vigilance and timely medical intervention. By understanding these complications, we can better advocate for prevention, early diagnosis, and comprehensive care to mitigate the impact of this serious illness.

How is Meningitis Diagnosed, and What Tests Are Commonly Used?

Diagnosing meningitis is a critical and urgent step in managing this potentially life-threatening condition. Early and accurate diagnosis not only facilitates timely treatment but also helps prevent severe complications. Given the varied causes and presentations of meningitis, the diagnostic process involves a combination of clinical evaluation, laboratory testing, and imaging techniques. These methods aim to identify the underlying cause of the inflammation, distinguish between bacterial, viral, fungal, and non-infectious meningitis, and assess the severity of the condition.

This chapter delves into the process of diagnosing meningitis, detailing the clinical signs, essential diagnostic tools, and the significance of each test in confirming the diagnosis and guiding treatment.

The Clinical Evaluation

The diagnostic journey for meningitis often begins with a detailed clinical evaluation. Physicians rely on a combination of patient history, physical examination, and symptom analysis to assess the likelihood of meningitis.

1. Patient History

A thorough medical history provides vital clues about potential risk factors and exposures. Key aspects include:

- **Recent illnesses:** Respiratory infections, ear infections, or sinusitis may precede bacterial meningitis.
- **Travel history:** Visits to regions with endemic diseases like meningococcal meningitis or parasitic infections can inform the diagnostic process.
- **Vaccination status:** Lack of vaccination against *Haemophilus influenzae* type b (Hib), pneumococcus, or meningococcus increases susceptibility.
- **Immune status:** Conditions like HIV/AIDS, recent chemotherapy, or organ transplantation can predispose individuals to fungal or opportunistic infections.

2. Physical Examination

The physical examination focuses on identifying hallmark signs of meningitis and assessing neurological function:

- **Neck stiffness:** Difficulty bending the neck forward is a classic symptom and can be tested using the Brudzinski and Kernig signs.

- **Skin examination:** A purpuric or petechial rash is often associated with meningococcal meningitis.
- **Neurological assessment:** Confusion, drowsiness, seizures, or focal neurological deficits signal CNS involvement.

While the clinical evaluation provides strong initial indications, definitive diagnosis requires laboratory and imaging studies to confirm meningitis and determine its cause.

Laboratory Testing for Meningitis

Laboratory testing is the cornerstone of meningitis diagnosis. These tests aim to detect the presence of pathogens, evaluate inflammatory markers, and analyze cerebrospinal fluid (CSF) composition.

1. Lumbar Puncture (Spinal Tap)

The lumbar puncture is the gold standard diagnostic test for meningitis. It involves extracting cerebrospinal fluid (CSF) from the spinal canal for analysis.

Procedure

- The patient is positioned lying on their side or sitting, and the lower back is cleaned and numbed.

- A thin, hollow needle is inserted between two vertebrae, typically in the lumbar region, to collect CSF.

CSF Analysis

CSF analysis provides critical information about the type and severity of meningitis:

- **Appearance:** Cloudy CSF often indicates bacterial meningitis, while clear CSF is more typical of viral meningitis.
- **Cell count:** Elevated white blood cell (WBC) counts suggest inflammation, with neutrophil predominance indicating bacterial meningitis and lymphocyte predominance suggesting viral or fungal causes.
- **Protein levels:** Increased protein levels reflect inflammation and disruption of the blood-brain barrier.
- **Glucose levels:** Reduced glucose levels are a hallmark of bacterial or fungal meningitis, as pathogens consume glucose.
- **Gram stain and culture:** A Gram stain provides a rapid assessment of bacterial presence, while cultures identify specific pathogens and their antibiotic susceptibilities.

2. Blood Cultures

Blood cultures are essential in diagnosing bacterial meningitis, as many cases involve bacteremia (bacteria in the bloodstream). By isolating and identifying the pathogen, blood cultures provide valuable information for targeted therapy.

- **Utility:** Blood cultures are especially useful in patients unable to undergo a lumbar puncture immediately.
- **Limitations:** Negative blood cultures do not rule out meningitis, as some pathogens may not be present in the bloodstream.

---

3. Polymerase Chain Reaction (PCR)

PCR is a molecular diagnostic tool that detects the genetic material of pathogens with high sensitivity and specificity.

- **Applications:** PCR is particularly valuable for identifying viral meningitis (e.g., enteroviruses, herpes simplex virus) and bacterial meningitis when Gram stain and cultures are inconclusive.
- **Advantages:** PCR can detect low levels of pathogens and identify non-culturable organisms.

- **Turnaround Time:** Results are often available within hours, aiding rapid diagnosis.

---

4. Serology

Serological tests detect antibodies or antigens in the blood or CSF. They are particularly useful for diagnosing fungal or parasitic meningitis.

- **Examples:** Cryptococcal antigen testing is highly sensitive for detecting *Cryptococcus neoformans*, a common cause of fungal meningitis.

---

5. Complete Blood Count (CBC) and Inflammatory Markers

Routine blood tests can provide additional clues about the severity of meningitis:

- **White blood cell count:** Elevated WBC counts suggest infection.
- **C-reactive protein (CRP) and procalcitonin:** These markers of inflammation are often elevated in bacterial meningitis and help differentiate it from viral causes.

Imaging Studies

Imaging studies, such as computed tomography
(CT) and magnetic resonance imaging (MRI), play
a supportive role in diagnosing meningitis. They are
particularly valuable for identifying complications
or contraindications to lumbar puncture.

1. Computed Tomography (CT)

A CT scan of the head is often performed before a
lumbar puncture to rule out conditions that may
increase the risk of brain herniation.

- **Indications:** CT is recommended for
  patients with focal neurological deficits,
  altered mental status, or a history of head
  trauma.
- **Findings:** While CT is not diagnostic of
  meningitis, it may reveal complications such
  as hydrocephalus, brain abscesses, or
  cerebral edema.

2. Magnetic Resonance Imaging (MRI)

MRI provides more detailed imaging than CT and is
useful for detecting subtle abnormalities.

- **Applications:** MRI is particularly valuable for identifying complications like infarctions, abscesses, or inflammation of the cranial nerves.
- **Findings:** MRI may show enhancement of the meninges, indicating inflammation.

Rapid Diagnostic Tests

In recent years, rapid diagnostic tests have been developed to facilitate the timely diagnosis of meningitis. These include:

- **Lateral flow assays:** These point-of-care tests can detect cryptococcal antigen within minutes.
- **Multiplex PCR panels:** These panels test for multiple pathogens simultaneously, reducing diagnostic delays.

Challenges in Diagnosing Meningitis

Despite advances in diagnostic technology, several challenges remain:

- **Atypical Presentations:** Infants, the elderly, and immunocompromised patients may exhibit subtle or non-classic symptoms.

- **Delays in Diagnosis:** Access to specialized tests, particularly in resource-limited settings, can delay treatment.
- **Non-Culturable Pathogens:** Some pathogens, such as viruses and certain bacteria, may not grow in standard cultures.

Case Studies

Case Study 1: Bacterial Meningitis in an Adult

A 45-year-old man presented with fever, severe headache, and confusion. On examination, he had neck stiffness and a purpuric rash. A lumbar puncture revealed cloudy CSF, elevated WBC count with neutrophil predominance, high protein levels, and low glucose levels. Gram stain showed gram-negative diplococci, confirming *Neisseria meningitidis*. Blood cultures corroborated the findings, and the patient was started on intravenous ceftriaxone, resulting in full recovery.

Case Study 2: Viral Meningitis in a Child

A 10-year-old child presented with fever, headache, and photophobia following a week of flu-like symptoms. CSF analysis revealed clear fluid, elevated WBC count with lymphocyte predominance, normal glucose, and mildly elevated protein levels. PCR testing identified enterovirus as the causative agent. The child was managed with supportive care and recovered within a week.

Advances in Meningitis Diagnosis

Ongoing research continues to improve the diagnostic landscape for meningitis:

- **Next-Generation Sequencing (NGS):** NGS allows comprehensive pathogen detection by analyzing the genetic material of all organisms in a sample.
- **Biomarker Discovery:** Novel biomarkers are being investigated to differentiate bacterial and viral meningitis with greater accuracy.

Meningitis diagnosis requires a multidisciplinary approach that combines clinical expertise, laboratory testing, and imaging. Each diagnostic tool plays a crucial role in unraveling the cause of meningitis and guiding appropriate treatment. Early and accurate diagnosis is the key to reducing morbidity and mortality, underscoring the importance of continued advancements in diagnostic technology.

What Are the Treatment Options for Different Types of Meningitis?

Meningitis is a serious condition that requires prompt and appropriate treatment to reduce its potentially life-threatening complications. The approach to treatment varies significantly depending on the type of meningitis—bacterial, viral, fungal, or other causes—as each has distinct pathogens, mechanisms, and clinical outcomes. Understanding the treatment options for each type is critical for managing the disease effectively and ensuring the best possible recovery.

This chapter explores the treatment modalities for meningitis, covering antibiotics, corticosteroids, antiviral and antifungal medications, immunosuppressants, and supportive care. It also highlights emerging therapies and the importance of individualized treatment strategies.

Treatment Overview

The goals of meningitis treatment are to:

1. Eradicate the underlying cause of the infection.

2. Alleviate inflammation and prevent complications.
3. Support the patient's overall health and recovery.

Early diagnosis is crucial, as delays in treatment—particularly for bacterial meningitis—can lead to severe outcomes. The choice of therapy depends on several factors, including the patient's age, immune status, suspected or confirmed causative agent, and the severity of the disease.

Treatment of Bacterial Meningitis

Bacterial meningitis is a medical emergency that requires immediate treatment. This type of meningitis is associated with high morbidity and mortality rates if not promptly addressed. The cornerstone of treatment includes **intravenous antibiotics** and **corticosteroids**.

1. Antibiotic Therapy

Antibiotics are the primary treatment for bacterial meningitis, targeting the specific bacteria responsible for the infection. Broad-spectrum antibiotics are often initiated empirically (before specific pathogens are identified) and later adjusted based on culture and sensitivity results.

- **Ceftriaxone or Cefotaxime:** These third-generation cephalosporins are highly effective against common pathogens like *Streptococcus pneumoniae* and *Neisseria meningitidis*.
- **Vancomycin:** Added when *penicillin-resistant* strains of *S. pneumoniae* are suspected.
- **Ampicillin:** Used to cover *Listeria monocytogenes*, particularly in newborns, older adults, and immunocompromised patients.
- **Meropenem or Chloramphenicol:** Alternatives for patients allergic to beta-lactams.

Duration of Antibiotic Therapy

- **7–14 days:** For meningitis caused by *N. meningitidis* or *H. influenzae*.
- **10–14 days:** For *S. pneumoniae*.
- **21 days or longer:** For *Listeria monocytogenes*.

2. Corticosteroids

Corticosteroids, such as dexamethasone, are used to reduce inflammation in the meninges and prevent complications like hearing loss or neurological damage.

Indications for Corticosteroids

- Recommended for bacterial meningitis caused by *S. pneumoniae* in adults and *H. influenzae* in children.
- Administered prior to or alongside the first dose of antibiotics for maximal effectiveness.

Limitations

- Corticosteroids are generally not recommended for neonates or for meningitis caused by *N. meningitidis* unless there are clear indications.

3. Supportive Care

- **Hydration:** Intravenous fluids help maintain electrolyte balance and prevent dehydration.
- **Oxygen therapy:** May be required for patients with respiratory distress.
- **Monitoring intracranial pressure:** Severe cases may necessitate interventions like ventricular drainage.

Treatment of Viral Meningitis

Viral meningitis, often referred to as aseptic meningitis, is generally less severe than bacterial meningitis. Most cases resolve on their own without specific treatment, but antiviral therapy and supportive care are crucial for certain types of viral infections.

1. Supportive Care

For the majority of viral meningitis cases, treatment focuses on alleviating symptoms and supporting the body's immune response.

Key Elements of Supportive Care

- **Rest:** Encourages recovery and helps reduce fatigue.
- **Hydration:** Oral or intravenous fluids to prevent dehydration.
- **Pain management:** Over-the-counter medications like acetaminophen or ibuprofen to reduce fever and alleviate headaches.

2. Antiviral Therapy

Antiviral medications are reserved for cases where specific viruses are identified or strongly suspected as the cause.

Common Antiviral Medications

- **Acyclovir:** Effective against herpes simplex virus (HSV) and varicella-zoster virus (VZV). Administered intravenously in severe cases.
- **Ganciclovir or Foscarnet:** Used for cytomegalovirus (CMV)-associated

meningitis, typically in
immunocompromised patients.

Duration of Antiviral Therapy

- HSV or VZV meningitis typically requires
  7–14 days of intravenous acyclovir.
- CMV-related cases may need prolonged
  treatment, depending on immune status.

3. Monitoring and Follow-Up

Patients recovering from viral meningitis should be
monitored for residual symptoms like headaches,
fatigue, or cognitive issues. Rarely, post-viral
complications such as chronic fatigue syndrome
may develop.

Treatment of Fungal Meningitis

Fungal meningitis is a rare but serious condition
that primarily affects immunocompromised
individuals. Treatment involves long-term
antifungal therapy tailored to the specific fungal
pathogen.

1. Antifungal Medications

Antifungal treatment is intensive and often requires
a combination of medications.

- **Amphotericin B:** A broad-spectrum antifungal often used as first-line therapy for *Cryptococcus neoformans* and other invasive fungi.
- **Fluconazole:** Used as a follow-up to amphotericin B or as a maintenance therapy for cryptococcal meningitis.
- **Voriconazole or Itraconazole:** Alternatives for specific fungal infections like aspergillosis.

Duration of Therapy

- **Induction phase:** 2–6 weeks of intravenous therapy with amphotericin B.
- **Consolidation and maintenance phases:** Several months of oral fluconazole to prevent recurrence.

2. Adjunctive Therapies

- **Intracranial pressure management:** Elevated intracranial pressure is common in fungal meningitis and may require therapeutic lumbar punctures or shunt placement.
- **Immune system support:** Optimizing immune function is critical, particularly in HIV-positive patients.

Treatment of Parasitic Meningitis

Parasitic meningitis, though rare, is often challenging to treat due to the limited availability of effective antiparasitic medications.

1. Medications

- **Miltefosine:** Used for *Naegleria fowleri* infections (primary amebic meningoencephalitis), although survival rates remain low.
- **Albendazole and Steroids:** Combined therapy for *Angiostrongylus cantonensis* (rat lungworm) infections.

2. Supportive Care

Supportive care, including management of seizures and intracranial pressure, is critical in all forms of parasitic meningitis.

Treatment of Non-Infectious Meningitis

Non-infectious meningitis results from conditions like autoimmune diseases, medications, or cancer. Treatment focuses on addressing the underlying cause and managing inflammation.

1. Immunosuppressants

Autoimmune-related meningitis may require corticosteroids, methotrexate, or biologics like rituximab to suppress inflammation.

2. Discontinuation of Offending Medications

Drug-induced meningitis often resolves upon stopping the medication responsible for triggering the condition.

3. Cancer-Associated Meningitis

For carcinomatous meningitis, treatment includes chemotherapy, radiation therapy, or targeted therapy based on the type of cancer.

Emerging Therapies and Advances

Advances in meningitis treatment continue to improve outcomes, particularly for severe and refractory cases.

1. Novel Antibiotics and Antivirals

The development of new antimicrobial agents aims to combat antibiotic-resistant bacteria and emerging viral pathogens.

2. Immunotherapies

Research into immunomodulators and vaccines holds promise for preventing and managing meningitis caused by rare or resistant pathogens.

3. Gene Therapy

Experimental gene therapies may offer solutions for certain forms of viral or genetic meningitis.

The Importance of Timely and Individualized Treatment

Effective treatment of meningitis depends on:

- **Rapid initiation of therapy:** Delays in treatment, especially for bacterial meningitis, increase the risk of complications and death.
- **Pathogen-specific treatment:** Identifying the causative agent is crucial for tailoring therapy.
- **Comprehensive care:** Managing symptoms and complications is essential for recovery.

Meningitis is a complex disease requiring a multifaceted treatment approach. From antibiotics and antifungals to supportive care and emerging therapies, the options are vast and continuously evolving. Timely diagnosis and appropriate treatment not only save lives but also reduce the long-term impact of this potentially devastating condition. As medical science progresses, the prospects for better outcomes and fewer complications continue to improve.

How Can Meningitis Be Prevented, and What Vaccines Are Available?

Prevention is the cornerstone of reducing the incidence and impact of meningitis, a potentially devastating disease. By adopting proactive measures, individuals and communities can significantly lower the risk of infection and its severe complications. Central to meningitis prevention are vaccination programs, which have transformed the public health landscape by drastically reducing cases caused by certain pathogens. Alongside vaccines, good hygiene practices, awareness, and targeted prophylactic measures play crucial roles in curbing the spread of meningitis.

In this chapter, we explore the various preventive strategies for meningitis, including a detailed look at available vaccines, their effectiveness, and the importance of immunization programs.
Additionally, we discuss the role of hygiene, public health interventions, and prophylactic antibiotics in mitigating the risks associated with this disease.

The Role of Prevention in Combating Meningitis

Prevention is especially critical in the context of meningitis due to its rapid progression and the potential for severe complications. Effective preventive strategies focus on:

1. **Reducing susceptibility:** Vaccines protect individuals by building immunity against specific pathogens.
2. **Interrupting transmission:** Hygiene and public health measures limit the spread of infectious agents.
3. **Protecting high-risk groups:** Prophylactic interventions safeguard individuals exposed to meningitis.

By understanding and implementing these strategies, communities can achieve significant reductions in meningitis-related morbidity and mortality.

Vaccination: The Frontline Defense Against Meningitis

Vaccination is the most effective tool for preventing certain types of meningitis. Vaccines work by priming the immune system to recognize and combat specific pathogens, reducing the likelihood of infection and its spread within populations.

1. Meningococcal Vaccines

Meningococcal meningitis, caused by *Neisseria meningitidis*, is a major global health concern, especially in regions like sub-Saharan Africa's "meningitis belt." Meningococcal vaccines target various serogroups of this bacterium.

Types of Meningococcal Vaccines

- **Meningococcal conjugate vaccines (MCV4):** Protect against serogroups A, C, W, and Y. Examples include MenACWY (Menactra, Menveo).
- **Meningococcal B vaccines (MenB):** Protect against serogroup B, a significant cause of meningitis in young adults. Examples include Bexsero and Trumenba.
- **Meningitis A vaccine (MenAfriVac):** Specifically designed for use in the African meningitis belt, where serogroup A was once a leading cause of outbreaks.

Vaccination Schedules

- **Routine vaccination:** Administered at 11–12 years of age, with a booster dose at 16 years.
- **High-risk groups:** Individuals in outbreak-prone areas, college students living in dormitories, military personnel, and travelers to endemic regions are advised to receive meningococcal vaccines.

Effectiveness

Meningococcal vaccines are highly effective, reducing the incidence of disease caused by the targeted serogroups by up to 90%.

2. Pneumococcal Vaccines

Streptococcus pneumoniae is a leading cause of bacterial meningitis, particularly in young children, older adults, and individuals with weakened immune systems. Pneumococcal vaccines provide protection against this pathogen.

Types of Pneumococcal Vaccines

- **Pneumococcal conjugate vaccine (PCV13):** Covers 13 strains of *S. pneumoniae* and is recommended for infants, young children, and certain adults.
- **Pneumococcal polysaccharide vaccine (PPSV23):** Covers 23 strains and is recommended for older adults and individuals with chronic medical conditions.

Vaccination Schedules

- **Children:** PCV13 is administered as a series of doses starting at 2 months of age.
- **Adults:** PPSV23 is recommended for adults aged 65 and older, with PCV13 given in certain high-risk cases.

Effectiveness

Pneumococcal vaccines have significantly reduced invasive pneumococcal diseases, including meningitis, with PCV13 achieving over 90% efficacy in preventing vaccine-type infections in children.

---

3. Haemophilus influenzae Type b (Hib) Vaccine

Haemophilus influenzae type b was once a leading cause of bacterial meningitis in children under five. The introduction of the Hib vaccine has led to a dramatic decline in cases worldwide.

Vaccination Schedule

- Administered as part of routine childhood immunizations at 2, 4, 6, and 12–15 months of age.

Effectiveness

The Hib vaccine is over 95% effective in preventing invasive diseases caused by *H. influenzae* type b.

---

4. Vaccines for Viral Causes of Meningitis

While no vaccines specifically target viral meningitis, several vaccines protect against viruses known to cause the disease.

Examples

- **Measles, Mumps, Rubella (MMR) Vaccine:** Protects against mumps, a significant cause of viral meningitis in unvaccinated populations.
- **Varicella Vaccine:** Prevents chickenpox and shingles, both of which can lead to meningitis caused by varicella-zoster virus.
- **Polio Vaccine:** Prevents poliovirus-associated meningitis.
- **Japanese Encephalitis Vaccine:** Recommended for travelers to endemic areas to prevent viral meningitis caused by Japanese encephalitis virus.

---

5. Vaccines for Fungal and Parasitic Meningitis

Currently, no vaccines are available for fungal or parasitic meningitis. Preventive strategies focus on reducing exposure to environmental sources and improving immune defenses.

Hygiene Practices and Public Health Measures

In addition to vaccination, adopting good hygiene practices and implementing public health measures can significantly reduce the risk of meningitis transmission.

1. Personal Hygiene

- **Handwashing:** Regular handwashing with soap and water is crucial for preventing the spread of viral and bacterial pathogens.
- **Respiratory etiquette:** Covering the mouth and nose while coughing or sneezing helps reduce the spread of respiratory droplets.

2. Avoiding Close Contact

- Avoiding close contact with individuals showing signs of respiratory infections reduces the risk of exposure to meningitis-causing pathogens.

3. Food Safety

- Properly washing and cooking food minimizes the risk of *Listeria monocytogenes*, a bacterium associated with meningitis.

Prophylactic Antibiotics for Close Contacts

When cases of bacterial meningitis are identified, prophylactic antibiotics may be administered to close contacts of the infected individual to prevent further spread.

1. Indications for Prophylaxis

Prophylactic antibiotics are recommended for:

- Household members and roommates of individuals with meningococcal meningitis.
- Healthcare workers exposed to respiratory secretions of an infected patient.

2. Commonly Used Antibiotics

- **Rifampin:** A short course of rifampin is often used for meningococcal meningitis.
- **Ciprofloxacin or Ceftriaxone:** These are alternatives, particularly for adults.

3. Timing

Prophylaxis is most effective when administered within 24 hours of exposure.

Preventing Outbreaks

Public health interventions are crucial for preventing meningitis outbreaks, particularly in high-risk settings like schools, colleges, and refugee camps.

1. Surveillance and Monitoring

- Early detection and reporting of cases enable rapid public health responses to contain outbreaks.

2. Mass Vaccination Campaigns

- During outbreaks, mass vaccination campaigns targeting the causative pathogen can help control the spread of disease.

The Importance of Education and Awareness

Educating the public about meningitis prevention, recognizing symptoms, and seeking timely medical care is essential for reducing disease burden.

Key Messages

- Ensure timely vaccination according to recommended schedules.

- Practice good hygiene to reduce exposure to infectious agents.
- Seek medical attention immediately for symptoms like severe headache, fever, and neck stiffness.

Case Studies: Prevention in Action

Case Study 1: Success of the MenAfriVac Campaign

The introduction of the MenAfriVac vaccine in Africa's meningitis belt has virtually eliminated serogroup A meningococcal meningitis, preventing hundreds of thousands of cases and deaths.

Case Study 2: Impact of the Hib Vaccine

In countries that have implemented routine Hib vaccination, cases of *Haemophilus influenzae* type b meningitis have declined by over 90%, showcasing the transformative impact of immunization.

Future Directions in Meningitis Prevention

Ongoing research aims to develop new vaccines and improve existing ones to broaden protection against meningitis-causing pathogens.

1. Multivalent Vaccines

- Development of vaccines that cover additional meningococcal serogroups, including serogroup X, which currently lacks a vaccine.

2. Universal Vaccines

- Efforts to create a universal meningitis vaccine targeting multiple bacterial, viral, and fungal pathogens.

3. Improved Delivery Systems

- Advances in vaccine delivery, such as needle-free devices and thermostable formulations, to increase accessibility in remote regions.

The prevention of meningitis hinges on a multi-faceted approach that combines vaccination, hygiene practices, prophylactic measures, and public health interventions. Vaccines remain the most powerful tool in reducing the global burden of meningitis, protecting millions from its devastating effects. By fostering awareness, improving access to vaccines, and supporting research into innovative preventive strategies, we can move closer to a world where meningitis is no longer a major public health threat.

Who Is Most at Risk for Meningitis, and What Are the Risk Factors?

Meningitis is a life-threatening condition that can affect anyone, but certain individuals and populations face a heightened risk due to specific factors. Recognizing these high-risk groups and understanding the circumstances that increase susceptibility are crucial for targeted prevention, early detection, and prompt treatment. This chapter explores the demographics, environments, and medical conditions that predispose individuals to meningitis and delves into the reasons behind their elevated vulnerability.

Overview of Risk Factors for Meningitis

Risk factors for meningitis can be broadly classified into the following categories:

1. **Age-related susceptibility**
2. **Environmental factors and living conditions**
3. **Medical and immunological factors**
4. **Behavioral and lifestyle factors**
5. **Regional and seasonal trends**

Each of these categories contributes to the overall risk, either by increasing exposure to meningitis-causing pathogens or by compromising the body's ability to fight infection.

---

1. Age-Related Susceptibility

Age is one of the most significant risk factors for meningitis, as it influences the development and function of the immune system. Certain age groups are disproportionately affected, with unique vulnerabilities and outcomes.

Infants and Young Children

Infants and young children, especially those under 5 years of age, are at the highest risk for meningitis. This is due to their immature immune systems and limited exposure to pathogens, making them less capable of fighting infections effectively.

Key Risk Factors

- **Immature immune defenses:** Newborns lack fully developed adaptive immunity, leaving them vulnerable to infections caused by pathogens like *Group B Streptococcus*, *Escherichia coli*, and *Haemophilus influenzae* type b (Hib).

- **Close contact with caregivers:** Frequent physical contact with caregivers can inadvertently expose infants to pathogens.
- **Premature birth:** Preterm infants are at an even higher risk due to underdeveloped immunity.

Impact of Vaccination

The introduction of vaccines like Hib, pneumococcal conjugate (PCV13), and meningococcal conjugate (MCV4) has significantly reduced the incidence of meningitis in children. However, unvaccinated or undervaccinated children remain vulnerable.

Adolescents and Young Adults

Adolescents and young adults, particularly those between 16 and 25 years of age, are at increased risk for meningococcal meningitis.

Key Risk Factors

- **Social behaviors:** Activities such as kissing, sharing drinks, and smoking can spread meningococcal bacteria.
- **Crowded living conditions:** College dormitories, military barracks, and shared accommodations facilitate the transmission of respiratory pathogens.

- **Decline in vaccine-induced immunity:**
  Immunity from childhood vaccinations may
  wane during adolescence, necessitating
  booster doses.

Older Adults

The risk of meningitis increases again in individuals
aged 65 and older due to the natural decline in
immune function (immunosenescence) and the
prevalence of chronic health conditions.

Key Risk Factors

- **Underlying illnesses:** Conditions like
  diabetes, chronic kidney disease, and cancer
  weaken the immune system, increasing
  susceptibility.
- **Malnutrition:** Nutritional deficiencies are
  more common in older adults and can impair
  immune responses.
- **Hospitalization and invasive procedures:**
  Older adults undergoing medical procedures
  are at risk for healthcare-associated
  meningitis caused by pathogens like
  Staphylococcus aureus.

---

2. Environmental Factors and Living Conditions

Certain environments and living conditions can amplify the risk of meningitis by facilitating the spread of infectious agents or exposing individuals to environmental pathogens.

Crowded Living Conditions

Crowded settings increase the likelihood of respiratory droplets spreading among individuals, making outbreaks more common.

High-Risk Populations

- **College students:** Shared dormitories and communal spaces create an ideal environment for meningococcal bacteria to spread.
- **Military personnel:** Close quarters in military barracks heighten the risk of meningococcal and other respiratory infections.
- **Prison populations:** Inmates are at increased risk due to overcrowding and limited access to healthcare.

Poor Sanitation

Inadequate sanitation contributes to the spread of pathogens like *Neisseria meningitidis*, enteroviruses, and *Cryptococcus*.

- Individuals in refugee camps or low-income communities where access to clean water and proper waste disposal is limited.

Seasonal and Regional Factors

- **Meningitis Belt:** Sub-Saharan Africa's "meningitis belt" experiences regular epidemics of meningococcal meningitis during the dry season, driven by low humidity, dust, and close human contact.
- **Seasonality in viral meningitis:** Enterovirus-associated meningitis peaks in late summer and early fall in temperate climates.

---

3. Medical and Immunological Factors

Certain medical conditions and treatments compromise the immune system, making individuals more susceptible to meningitis.

Immunocompromised Individuals

Weakened immunity, whether due to underlying illness or medical treatments, significantly increases the risk of meningitis.

- **HIV/AIDS:** Individuals with advanced HIV infection are at risk for opportunistic meningitis caused by *Cryptococcus neoformans* and other pathogens.
- **Cancer and chemotherapy:** Treatments that suppress bone marrow function reduce the production of immune cells.
- **Organ transplantation:** Immunosuppressive drugs given to prevent organ rejection increase vulnerability to fungal and viral meningitis.

Splenectomy or Asplenia

The spleen plays a crucial role in filtering bacteria from the bloodstream. Individuals who have had their spleen removed or have nonfunctional spleens (as in sickle cell disease) are at increased risk for infections caused by encapsulated bacteria like *Streptococcus pneumoniae*, *Neisseria meningitidis*, and *Haemophilus influenzae*.

Chronic Conditions

Chronic illnesses such as diabetes, cirrhosis, and kidney disease impair immune responses and increase the risk of meningitis.

Head Trauma and Neurosurgical Procedures

- **Skull fractures:** Trauma that disrupts the meninges provides a direct pathway for bacteria to enter the cerebrospinal fluid (CSF).
- **Neurosurgery:** Procedures like ventricular shunting can introduce pathogens into the central nervous system, leading to healthcare-associated meningitis.

4. Behavioral and Lifestyle Factors

Certain behaviors and lifestyle choices can increase the likelihood of exposure to meningitis-causing pathogens.

Smoking

Smoking damages the respiratory tract, making it easier for bacteria like *Neisseria meningitidis* to colonize and invade the bloodstream.

Substance Abuse

Intravenous drug use introduces pathogens directly into the bloodstream, increasing the risk of bacterial meningitis.

Travel and Occupational Risks

- **Travel to endemic areas:** Travelers to regions like the meningitis belt in Africa are at heightened risk for meningococcal meningitis.
- **Healthcare workers:** Exposure to infectious agents in clinical settings places healthcare workers at risk, particularly during meningitis outbreaks.

---

5. Newborns and Perinatal Risk Factors

Newborns are particularly vulnerable to meningitis due to factors related to childbirth and early life.

Maternal Factors

- **Group B Streptococcus (GBS) colonization:** Mothers who carry GBS can transmit the bacteria to their newborns during delivery.

- **Prolonged rupture of membranes:**
  Increases the risk of neonatal exposure to
  pathogens like GBS and *Escherichia coli*.

Preventing Meningitis in High-Risk Groups

Preventive measures tailored to high-risk groups
can significantly reduce the incidence of meningitis.

1. Vaccination

- Routine childhood immunizations protect
  infants and children.
- Booster doses for adolescents and young
  adults maintain immunity.
- Targeted vaccination campaigns in
  outbreak-prone areas prevent epidemics.

2. Hygiene and Sanitation

- Handwashing, respiratory etiquette, and safe
  food practices reduce the spread of
  pathogens.

3. Prophylactic Antibiotics

- Administered to close contacts of individuals with bacterial meningitis to prevent secondary cases.

---

4. Public Health Interventions

- Surveillance systems monitor and respond to outbreaks.
- Education campaigns raise awareness about meningitis symptoms and prevention.

Meningitis disproportionately affects certain populations due to age, environmental factors, and underlying health conditions. By identifying high-risk groups and understanding the associated risk factors, we can implement targeted interventions to protect vulnerable individuals and reduce the overall burden of this serious disease.

What Public Health Strategies Are Used to Control Meningitis Outbreaks?

Meningitis outbreaks represent a significant public health challenge, particularly in regions where healthcare resources are limited, and preventive measures are not widely implemented. The rapid progression of meningitis and its potential for high mortality and long-term complications demand prompt and effective public health strategies to mitigate its impact. From mass vaccination campaigns to public awareness initiatives, controlling meningitis outbreaks involves a coordinated approach that integrates prevention, early detection, and rapid response.

This chapter explores the various public health measures employed to manage meningitis outbreaks, focusing on mass vaccination, community education, disease surveillance, and response protocols. By understanding these strategies, we can appreciate the global efforts to reduce the burden of meningitis and protect vulnerable populations.

The Scope of Meningitis Outbreaks

Meningitis outbreaks can occur sporadically or in large epidemics, with certain regions and populations at higher risk. The sub-Saharan African "meningitis belt," stretching from Senegal to Ethiopia, is particularly prone to meningococcal meningitis outbreaks, often triggered by climatic and social factors. However, meningitis outbreaks can occur anywhere, underscoring the importance of global vigilance.

Key Characteristics of Meningitis Outbreaks

1. **High Mortality Rates:** Without prompt treatment, bacterial meningitis can have a fatality rate of up to 50%.
2. **Rapid Spread:** Close contact, crowded conditions, and delayed recognition facilitate the transmission of meningitis-causing pathogens.
3. **Potential for Long-Term Disabilities:** Survivors often face complications such as hearing loss, cognitive impairment, or neurological deficits.

1. Mass Vaccination Campaigns

Vaccination is the cornerstone of meningitis outbreak control, particularly for bacterial meningitis caused by *Neisseria meningitidis*,

Haemophilus influenzae type b, and *Streptococcus pneumoniae*. Mass vaccination campaigns aim to immunize large populations quickly to interrupt transmission and prevent further cases.

A. Targeted Vaccination During Outbreaks

In outbreak scenarios, public health authorities prioritize vaccinating at-risk populations, including:

- Close contacts of confirmed cases.
- Residents of outbreak-prone areas.
- Vulnerable groups such as children, adolescents, and immunocompromised individuals.

B. MenAfriVac Success in the African Meningitis Belt

The MenAfriVac vaccine, developed to target *Neisseria meningitidis* serogroup A, has revolutionized meningitis control in Africa. Introduced in 2010, it has virtually eliminated serogroup A meningitis in the meningitis belt.

Implementation Highlights

- Mass immunization campaigns reached over 350 million people within a decade.
- Vaccination coverage exceeded 80% in most target regions, leading to a dramatic decline in cases.

C. Routine Immunization Programs

Incorporating meningitis vaccines into routine immunization schedules helps prevent outbreaks by maintaining population immunity. Key vaccines include:

- Meningococcal conjugate vaccines (MCV4).
- Pneumococcal conjugate vaccines (PCV13).
- Haemophilus influenzae type b (Hib) vaccines.

---

2. Public Awareness and Community Education

Public awareness is a critical component of meningitis outbreak control. Educating communities about the symptoms, transmission, and prevention of meningitis encourages early medical attention and reduces stigma associated with the disease.

A. Community Engagement

Public health authorities often partner with community leaders, educators, and religious figures to disseminate information effectively. Strategies include:

- **Workshops and seminars:** Local gatherings to explain meningitis prevention and treatment.
- **Media campaigns:** Radio, television, and social media platforms are used to spread awareness.
- **School programs:** Children are educated about hygiene practices and the importance of vaccination.

B. Recognizing Symptoms

Teaching communities to recognize the early signs of meningitis—such as fever, headache, neck stiffness, and sensitivity to light—can facilitate timely medical intervention, reducing morbidity and mortality.

3. Disease Surveillance and Early Detection

Effective surveillance systems are essential for identifying meningitis outbreaks early and initiating a rapid response. Surveillance involves monitoring disease trends, detecting clusters of cases, and identifying causative pathogens.

A. Sentinel Surveillance Systems

In many regions, sentinel surveillance systems collect data from designated healthcare facilities to track meningitis cases. This data helps:

- Detect outbreaks in their early stages.
- Identify the serogroups or pathogens involved.
- Guide vaccination and treatment strategies.

B. Laboratory Diagnostics

Laboratories play a vital role in confirming meningitis cases and determining the causative agent. Key diagnostic tools include:

- Lumbar puncture for cerebrospinal fluid (CSF) analysis.
- Polymerase chain reaction (PCR) for pathogen identification.
- Serological tests to detect specific antigens or antibodies.

C. Real-Time Data Sharing

Advancements in technology have enabled real-time data sharing between healthcare facilities and public health authorities, improving outbreak detection and response times.

4. Rapid Response Protocols

Once an outbreak is identified, rapid response protocols are activated to contain the spread and minimize the impact. These protocols involve a coordinated effort between healthcare providers, government agencies, and international organizations.

A. Outbreak Investigation

Public health teams investigate the outbreak to determine:

- The extent of the outbreak and affected populations.
- The causative pathogen and its antibiotic susceptibility.
- The potential sources of infection and modes of transmission.

B. Emergency Mass Vaccination

Emergency vaccination campaigns are launched in response to outbreaks, targeting unvaccinated or at-risk populations.

C. Antibiotic Prophylaxis

Close contacts of confirmed cases are provided with prophylactic antibiotics, such as rifampin or ciprofloxacin, to prevent secondary cases.

D. Case Management

Healthcare facilities are mobilized to provide:

- Immediate treatment for suspected and confirmed cases.

- Supportive care, including hydration and oxygen therapy.
- Management of complications like seizures or hydrocephalus.

---

5. International Collaboration in Outbreak Control

Meningitis outbreaks often cross borders, requiring international collaboration for effective management. Organizations like the World Health Organization (WHO) and Médecins Sans Frontières (MSF) play crucial roles in coordinating global responses.

A. WHO Epidemic Response Guidelines

The WHO provides technical support and resources to countries facing meningitis outbreaks, including:

- Guidelines for case management and vaccination strategies.
- Stockpiles of meningitis vaccines for emergency use.

B. The Global Meningitis Initiative

This coalition of health organizations works to eliminate meningitis as a public health threat by:

- Promoting vaccine access and affordability.

- Supporting research into new prevention and treatment strategies.

C. Cross-Border Cooperation

Neighboring countries collaborate to:

- Share surveillance data and laboratory resources.
- Coordinate vaccination campaigns in border regions.

Case Studies: Success Stories in Meningitis Outbreak Control

Case Study 1: MenAfriVac in the African Meningitis Belt

The introduction of the MenAfriVac vaccine has transformed meningitis control in Africa, reducing cases of serogroup A meningitis by over 99%.

Case Study 2: Public Health Response in New Zealand

During a meningococcal B outbreak in the early 2000s, New Zealand implemented a targeted vaccination program, achieving high coverage and effectively halting the outbreak.

Challenges in Meningitis Outbreak Control

Despite advancements, several challenges remain:

- **Vaccine accessibility:** High costs and logistical barriers limit vaccine availability in low-income countries.
- **Emerging serogroups:** Pathogens like *Neisseria meningitidis* serogroup X currently lack effective vaccines.
- **Antibiotic resistance:** Rising resistance complicates treatment and prophylaxis efforts.

Future Directions in Meningitis Outbreak Prevention

Advances in technology and research offer hope for more effective meningitis control strategies in the future.

A. Development of Universal Vaccines

Efforts are underway to create a universal meningitis vaccine that protects against all major bacterial serogroups.

B. Enhanced Surveillance Systems

Integration of artificial intelligence and big data analytics into surveillance systems promises to improve outbreak detection and response.

C. Community-Based Interventions

Innovative approaches, such as mobile vaccination units and community health worker programs, aim to increase coverage in remote and underserved areas.

Controlling meningitis outbreaks requires a comprehensive public health strategy that combines vaccination, community engagement, surveillance, and rapid response. Success stories like the MenAfriVac campaign demonstrate the power of coordinated efforts in reducing the burden of this devastating disease. As global health initiatives continue to evolve, the vision of a world free from meningitis outbreaks becomes increasingly attainable.

What is the Prognosis for Individuals Diagnosed with Meningitis, and How Does it Vary by Type?

Meningitis is a severe condition that requires prompt recognition and treatment to improve outcomes. While advancements in medical care have significantly increased survival rates, the prognosis for individuals diagnosed with meningitis varies widely depending on several factors. These factors include the type of meningitis (bacterial, viral, fungal, or parasitic), the patient's age, underlying health status, and how quickly treatment is initiated. The outcomes can range from full recovery to severe long-term complications or, in some cases, death.

This chapter explores the prognosis of meningitis, examining the factors that influence recovery and survival. We will also delve into the distinctions between the types of meningitis and how they affect patient outcomes.

Understanding Prognosis in Meningitis

The prognosis of meningitis refers to the likely outcome of the disease and the patient's ability to recover fully or partially. This depends on:

1. **Severity and type of meningitis**: Some forms, like bacterial meningitis, are more aggressive and have higher mortality rates than viral or fungal meningitis.
2. **Timeliness of diagnosis and treatment**: Early treatment is critical to reducing the risk of complications.
3. **Patient demographics**: Age, overall health, and preexisting conditions play significant roles in determining recovery.

Prognosis by Type of Meningitis

The type of meningitis is the most significant determinant of prognosis. Each type presents unique challenges and outcomes based on its causative agent and how it affects the body.

1. Bacterial Meningitis

Bacterial meningitis is the most severe form of meningitis, with a high risk of death and long-term complications if not treated promptly. However, with early and effective treatment, the prognosis improves significantly.

Mortality Rates

- **Without treatment:** Mortality rates can be as high as 50%.

- **With treatment:** Mortality decreases to 10–15%, depending on the pathogen and the patient's condition.

Long-Term Complications

Even with treatment, bacterial meningitis can leave survivors with lasting effects:

- **Neurological deficits**: Cognitive impairments, memory problems, or difficulties with concentration.
- **Hearing loss**: Damage to the auditory nerves is common, especially in children.
- **Seizures**: Brain damage from inflammation can lead to epilepsy in some cases.
- **Motor impairments**: Paralysis or weakness due to brain or nerve damage.

Prognosis by Pathogen

- **Streptococcus pneumoniae**: Associated with a higher risk of death and long-term complications, particularly in older adults.
- **Neisseria meningitidis**: Rapid progression can lead to fatal outcomes without treatment, but survivors generally recover well if treated promptly.
- **Haemophilus influenzae type b (Hib)**: Prognosis has improved dramatically with widespread vaccination, although complications can still occur in unvaccinated individuals.

- **Listeria monocytogenes**: Prognosis is poorer in neonates, pregnant women, and immunocompromised individuals.

2. Viral Meningitis

Viral meningitis, also known as aseptic meningitis, generally has a more favorable prognosis than bacterial meningitis. Most cases resolve without specific treatment, although the recovery timeline varies.

Recovery

- **Mild cases**: Recovery typically occurs within 7–10 days.
- **Severe cases**: Some individuals may experience lingering symptoms, such as fatigue, headaches, or memory problems, for weeks or months.

Complications

While rare, complications can include:

- **Chronic headaches**: Persistent headaches that may require long-term management.
- **Cognitive effects**: Temporary difficulties with memory or concentration.
- **Seizures**: In severe cases, particularly with herpes simplex virus (HSV) or other neurotropic viruses.

- **Enteroviruses**: The most common cause of viral meningitis, associated with excellent recovery rates.
- **Herpes simplex virus (HSV)**: Can cause severe encephalitis, leading to neurological deficits if not treated promptly.
- **Varicella-zoster virus (VZV)**: Generally resolves well with antiviral treatment, although complications may arise in immunocompromised individuals.

---

3. Fungal Meningitis

Fungal meningitis is a serious condition that primarily affects immunocompromised individuals. The prognosis depends on the pathogen, the patient's immune status, and the timeliness of treatment.

Mortality Rates

- Mortality is high without treatment, ranging from 40–80%.
- With early antifungal therapy, mortality rates drop significantly, but the disease still carries a high risk of complications.

- **Neurological impairments**: Chronic inflammation can lead to cognitive and motor deficits.
- **Hydrocephalus**: Increased intracranial pressure may require surgical intervention.
- **Relapse**: Recurrence is common, particularly in patients with ongoing immune suppression.

Prognosis by Pathogen

- **Cryptococcus neoformans**: Common in HIV/AIDS patients; outcomes are improved with amphotericin B and fluconazole therapy.
- **Candida species**: Often associated with hospital-acquired infections; prognosis depends on early detection and aggressive treatment.

---

4. Parasitic Meningitis

Parasitic meningitis is rare but often fatal, particularly when caused by organisms like *Naegleria fowleri* (primary amebic meningoencephalitis).

Mortality Rates

- *Naegleria fowleri*: Nearly 100% fatal without treatment; even with treatment, survival rates are less than 5%.
- Other parasitic infections, such as those caused by *Angiostrongylus cantonensis* (rat lungworm), have better outcomes if treated early.

Complications

- Neurological damage is common in survivors, including seizures and cognitive deficits.

Factors Influencing Prognosis

Several factors contribute to the prognosis of meningitis, influencing both survival and the risk of long-term complications.

1. Timeliness of Diagnosis and Treatment

Early diagnosis and prompt initiation of treatment are critical for improving outcomes.

- **Delays in treatment**: Lead to higher mortality rates and a greater likelihood of complications.
- **Immediate care**: Antibiotics for bacterial meningitis or antivirals for viral causes can drastically improve survival.

2. Age

- **Infants and young children**: Higher risk of severe disease and long-term complications due to immature immune systems.
- **Older adults**: Increased mortality and complications due to comorbidities and weaker immune responses.

3. Immune Status

- Immunocompromised individuals are more likely to experience severe disease and poor outcomes.

4. Pathogen Virulence

- Highly virulent pathogens like *Neisseria meningitidis* and *Naegleria fowleri* are associated with worse outcomes.

5. Access to Medical Care

- Regions with limited healthcare infrastructure face higher mortality rates and long-term disabilities due to delayed or inadequate treatment.

Improving Prognosis: Key Strategies

Efforts to improve the prognosis of meningitis focus on prevention, early detection, and advancements in treatment.

1. Vaccination

- Routine immunization programs have drastically reduced the incidence of meningitis caused by Hib, pneumococcus, and meningococcus.

2. Early Diagnosis

- Improved diagnostic tools, such as polymerase chain reaction (PCR) and rapid antigen tests, facilitate early detection and tailored treatment.

3. Comprehensive Care

- Multidisciplinary approaches, including neurology, rehabilitation, and psychological support, help manage long-term complications.

4. Public Awareness

- Educating communities about meningitis symptoms and the importance of seeking medical care early can improve outcomes.

Case Studies: Prognosis in Real-World Scenarios

Case Study 1: Meningococcal Meningitis in a College Student

A 19-year-old college student presented with fever, severe headache, and a purpuric rash. Diagnosis of *Neisseria meningitidis* was confirmed, and intravenous antibiotics were initiated within hours. The patient recovered fully within two weeks, highlighting the importance of early treatment and robust healthcare infrastructure.

Case Study 2: Cryptococcal Meningitis in an HIV Patient

A 35-year-old man with advanced HIV/AIDS was diagnosed with cryptococcal meningitis. Despite aggressive antifungal therapy, he experienced hydrocephalus and required a ventriculoperitoneal shunt. Long-term maintenance therapy with fluconazole prevented recurrence.

The prognosis of meningitis varies widely based on the type of meningitis, the timeliness of treatment, and the patient's individual risk factors. While bacterial meningitis carries the highest risk of mortality and long-term complications, prompt treatment can significantly improve outcomes. Viral meningitis generally has a favorable prognosis, while fungal and parasitic forms pose greater challenges due to their association with immunocompromised individuals.

Advances in vaccination, diagnostic techniques, and treatment protocols have improved survival rates and reduced complications in many cases. However, continued efforts are needed to address disparities in access to care and to develop effective strategies for managing rare and severe forms of meningitis. By focusing on prevention, early detection, and comprehensive care, we can enhance the prognosis for individuals diagnosed with this serious condition.

Thank You for Reading

Dear Reader,

Thank you for reading the book. If you enjoyed this book or found it useful, I'd be very grateful if you'd post a short review. Your support really does make a difference, and I read all the reviews personally so I can get your feedback and make this book even better. If this book resonated with you or inspired new perspectives, please consider supporting future projects and publications. Your generous contributions make it possible to continue creating meaningful content.

Support My Work:

Venmo: @Nileshlp
Cash App: $drnileshlp

BTC

bc1qs72228z6pauw3rk9tej9f6umu4y9gz289y3cvn

ETH

0xE1DAE6F656c900a4b24257b587ac0856E1e346D2

Every bit of support goes a long way in sustaining my passion for storytelling and public health advocacy. Once again, thank you from the bottom of my heart. Your encouragement and generosity mean the world to me.

Warm regards,
Dr. Nilesh Panchal
Author and Public Health Practitioner

Printed in Dunstable, United Kingdom